JOCELINE KING

SUPPLEMENT HANDBOOK

The Ultimate Guide to Health Supplements, Learn All the Information About Different Dietary Supplements That Can Help You Get and Stay Healthy

Descrierea CIP a Bibliotecii Naţionale a României
JOCELINE KING
    **SUPPLEMENT HANDBOOK. The Ultimate Guide to
Health Supplements, Learn All the Information About
Different Dietary Supplements That Can Help You Get and
Stay Healthy** / Joceline King – Bucharest: Editura My Ebook, 2020
    ISBN

JOCELINE KING

SUPPLEMENT HANDBOOK

The Ultimate Guide to Health Supplements, Learn All the Information About Different Dietary Supplements That Can Help You Get and Stay Healthy

My Ebook Publishing House
Bucharest, 2020

CONTENTS

1

SUPPLEMENTS FOR HEALTH

VITAMIN MYTHS

When checking out facts about Vitamin B, it is important to be able to differentiate between what information is an actual fact, and what is simply a myth. Unfortunately, there are myths about just about everything, so any information learned on any topic should always be evaluated before deciding whether or not it is true. There are many myths about vitamins and supplements in circulation today. Some vitamins, such as vitamin D, have many myths attributed to their use. Others, such as vitamin A, do not have any at all. The following sections will break down the myths about specific vitamins.

VITAMIN B

A common rumor is that the B complex vitamins, including Folic acid will reduce the risk of heart disease in women who are prone to heart problems. This theory has been tested, and is proven to be false. Studies show that women who took B complex vitamins and Folic acid were no less likely to have heart problems than women who did not consume these supplements.

Some say that Vitamin B-1, which is also called thiamine, helps with the growth of hair at the roots. You will even hear that the hair will not grow properly without this vitamin. Some rumors are even passed around that claim Vitamin B-1 assists with the root development of plants as well. This is certainly not the case, as there are no scientific studies to back up such claims. Another version of this rumor is that taking Vitamin B-1 helps to reduce transplant shock for either people who are receiving new organs, or plants that are being moved. Again, this is not at all the case.

Have you been told that Vitamin B-6 is safe for you to consume, even if it is taken above the recommended limit? This is supposedly true, because it is a water-soluble vitamin. However, the myth is also quite false, as excessive B-6 in the human body can lead to neuropathy pain, skin lesions, vomiting, and even more health problems. Vitamin B-6, like any other vitamin, is best taken within the recommended dosages. Another rumor about vitamin B-6 is that it is an effective treatment for PMS. While double-blind studies were done that initially proved this to be the case, further analysis of those studies have proven them to be inaccurate.

Vitamin B-12 is received by most individuals through the ingestion of meat. Vegans and vegetarians, however do not get this vitamin from eating meat, for obvious reasons! This fact lends credence to the myth that people need B-12 every day in high dosages. In truth, B-12 is needed in exceptionally small amounts, only about 2 micrograms a day, as the body can store up years worth of B-12 for future use. For this reason, going without this vitamin is not usually problematic as long as it is ingested occasionally in one form or another.

VITAMIN C
While Vitamin C is quite good for you, and does help to build the immune system, taking a huge dose of vitamin C will not keep a cold away! Scientists have cured many illnesses, as you know. However, as the old saying goes, there is no cure for the common cold! Vitamin C is no miracle cure for any illness,

sadly. There have never been any scientific studies done that would prove otherwise.

VITAMIN D

One very interesting myth about Vitamin D is contained in its moniker! You see, Vitamin D is not actually a vitamin. While it is quite essential to the body, and for this reason is referred to as one, Vitamin D is actually a hormone!

As it is commonly known, Vitamin D is made in the body by sun exposure. This is a true fact, however it is a myth to believe that a sufficient amount of vitamin D can be gained in the body simply by normal day-to-day exposure to the sun. Unless someone spends large amounts of time outdoors, most people do not get enough sunshine in their everyday lives to produce the required amount of vitamin D. Purposely sunning to try and avoid Vitamin D deficiency is definitely not a good idea! In order for your skin to absorb the sun's rays, you would have to go out in the sun unprotected by sunscreen. Instead of preventing a deficiency, this could very likely cause skin cancer.

The next myth is that the proper level of Vitamin D can be sufficiently gained through diet. This is incorrect, as the body naturally produces Vitamin D-3. Food sold in supermarkets generally contains Vitamin D-2 when the label states that the
12

product has Vitamin D. In fact, in addition to this statement, recent studies show that the amount of Vitamin D listed on the labels of most foods is completely inaccurate more than half of the time!

Another myth regarding Vitamin D is that it should be avoided by pregnant and breastfeeding women. Regardless of whether or not you are pregnant, it is encouraged that all individuals receive 400 IU of Vitamin D on a daily basis. Babies should receive 210 IU of Vitamin D each day. Since Vitamin D crosses over into the breast milk, it is better to make sure the mother receives 4,000 IU of vitamin D instead of supplementing the child's diet.

VITAMIN E

Perhaps the most commonly believed myth about Vitamin E is that it helps to heal wounds, and can also decrease scars on the skin. Studies have shown that Vitamin E has no positive effects on scars or wounds, and in fact can even be bad for the skin. Vitamin E has a tendency to prove rather irritating to the skin, and can even cause an allergic reaction. When used on burn scars, for example, Vitamin E has been shown to cause the scars to become more discolored than they were before!

LITTLE KNOWN FACTS ABOUT VITAMINS

VITAMIN A

While most people know that Vitamin A is needed for the body's good health, they do not realize what happens when the supplement is taken in excess. Too much Vitamin A can actually cause liver damage, damage to the nervous system, yellow skin, hair loss, and bone damage. In pregnant women, excess Vitamin A can cause birth defects to the child.

If you take it in the correct amounts, Vitamin A is not only healthy, but is also known to be essential to most bodily functions. The best way to get enough Vitamin A is through the foods you eat. This important vitamin can be found naturally in eggs, whole milk, liver, and in fruits and vegetables that are brightly colored.

Vitamin A is absolutely essential because when it is not received by the body in adequate proportions, it can lead to immunity problems and infections. Luckily, this is rather uncommon in developed countries, and usually is only problematic with those who are on strict diets or maintain a high alcohol intake.

VITAMIN B

Vitamin B is actually a group of four vitamins, vitamin B-1 also called thiamine, vitamin B-2 also called riboflavin, vitamin B-6 also called pyridoxine, and vitamin B-12 also called cobalamin. Together, these four vitamins make the B vitamin group.

Most individuals in developed countries get plenty of B vitamins; however vegetarians sometimes have a deficiency due to their being found primarily in animals. Some medications also affect the way B vitamins are absorbed into the body and can cause a deficiency. A vitamin B deficiency is usually characterized by skin rashes, nerve problems, and anemia.

Although a B vitamin overdose is almost unheard of, when it does occur symptoms include severe burning of any part of the body, itching, or numbness. As with all supplements, it is best to take vitamin B only as recommended.

VITAMIN C

Ascorbic Acid, which is another name for Vitamin C, is essential for helping the body absorb iron. When too much Vitamin C is taken, it can cause diarrhea and stomach pain. This is important to keep in mind when someone suggests taking a Vitamin C overload to help cure a cold!

Vitamin C is has been commonly associated with the immune system. What most people do not realize, however, is that there is a whole host of potential problems that can come from a deficiency of Vitamin C. Lesser known problems stemming from a lack of Vitamin C include nosebleeds, general weakness and lassitude, swollen gums, and scurvy.

Vitamin C is found naturally in most fruits and vegetables, and is found in larger portions in raspberries, cantaloupe, broccoli, strawberries, and cabbage. Surprisingly, Vitamin C can also be found in liver. When taken in the form of supplements, Vitamin C is best consumed in liquid form, as the pill form is not always absorbed properly by the body.

VITAMIN D

There are actually two different forms of vitamin D. There is one form that is found in vegetables, and another form found in animals. The form of Vitamin D found in vegetables is called ergocalciferol, while the alternative form is called cholecalciferol. This is the form that is metabolized by the body whenever we expose it to sunlight.

Vitamin D is an essential hormone in the body, and deficiencies are usually found in people who have milk allergies, lactose intolerance, or those who are strict vegetarians. When not enough Vitamin D is taken into the body, it can cause rickets and osteomalacia, which are both diseases that affect the bone structure.

When too much Vitamin D is consumed, however, it can cause an over- absorption of calcium. This can result in calcification, urinary stones, and problems with the central nervous system. Problems with the central muscle system can show up as well. Vitamin D should be taken only as recommended by your doctor.

VITAMIN E

Vitamin E is found in wheat germ, spinach, olives, nuts, seeds, and leafy greens. Eating foods that are rich in Vitamin E can help to prevent Alzheimer's disease and prostate cancer, as well as helping to guard against the UV rays of the sun.

Although it is exceptionally rare for people to develop a Vitamin E deficiency, it's still important to make sure that the recommended daily dose is taken. A Vitamin E deficiency has been known to cause severe problems with the nervous system.

Too much Vitamin E can cause fatigue, weakness, flu-like symptoms, abdominal pain, internal bleeding, and headaches. These symptoms will increase in severity if the overdose is continued over a period of time.

2

VITAMINS AND KIDS

SHOULD CHILDREN TAKE VITAMINS?

Over the years, there has been much controversy over whether or not children should take vitamins. It is the opinion of some that the necessary vitamins can be taken in through a proper diet that has a good nutritional balance. Unfortunately, this is not always the case in today's busy world. Vitamins that are found naturally in many foods have been depleted of much of their nutritional value by being processed, frozen, and cooked. Vitamins are important for the health of all people, but especially important for growing children.

ARE THERE POSSIBLE DANGERS?

There are very few dangers to giving children vitamins. The biggest dangers actually come from mismanagement of vitamins. While quite healthy for the body in the proper amounts, it is never good to exceed the recommended dosage of vitamins, especially in children. With the variety of candy colored, cartoon character shaped chewable vitamins available for kids, it's important that the bottle containing them is stored well out of the reach of children. Often, children will think that their daily multi-vitamin is candy, and will want to take more than one, especially if they can sneak a few out of the bottle without Mom knowing!. An overdose of vitamins can cause a vast variety of health problems and other symptoms as well as long term damage to vital organs.

Overdoses of most vitamins are almost unheard of, and are avoidable simply by following the instructions on the bottle. It is never a good idea to increase the dose of vitamins you are taking past the recommended limit unless you are instructed to do so by your doctor for some medically necessary reason. More often than not, the opposite will be true, where children risk growing up without the full dose of essential vitamins.

WHAT IF A CHILD OVERDOSES ON VITAMINS?

In the event of an overdose on vitamins, children can experience a vast array of symptoms. These symptoms can include but are not limited to stomach pain, nausea, diarrhea, headaches, and dizziness. In more severe cases, iron toxicity, stomach bleeding, and heart damage can be seen.

When someone experiences an accidental overdose, it is essential for them to seek medical attention for them immediately. This necessity may fall on the shoulders of a friend or relative of this person The best possible course of action, however, would be to avoid overdose completely. Simple precautions can be taken by keeping vitamins out of the reach of children and the elderly. You can administer the vitamins to the family each day in order to monitor the dosages. As the old saying goes, an ounce of prevention is worth a pound of cure.

WHAT EFFECTS DO VITAMINS HAVE ON CHILDREN?

Vitamins have a number of different effects on children. Physically, vitamins allow children to grow and develop properly. A proper balance of vitamins will produce children with bones and muscles that will stay strong, and also will help to improve vision, coordination, and motor skills.

Vitamins also greatly affect the way children are able to learn. Vitamins are essential to brain development, and contribute to the ability to take in, comprehend, process, and store knowledge. A correct balance of vitamins has also been shown to improve the ability a child has to focus and concentrate. With children spending seven hours a day in school and quite a few hours on homework once returning home, vitamins are quite important for keeping children on task.

LONG TERM EFFECTS

For those individuals who received all of the necessary vitamins as small children, and continued this practice through their adulthood, there are many satisfactory long term effects.

Adults who have grown up receiving the proper balance of vitamins their entire lives have better vision, sharper memories, a decreased chance of developing Alzheimer's disease, bone and joint problems, and/or osteoporosis.

WHAT SHOULD CHILDREN TAKE?

With all the vitamins available on today's market, it can be difficult to decide what kind of vitamins to give a child. While the following will give you a comprehensive guide to what the average child needs, it is always best to consult a doctor on the specific needs of your individual child.

INDIVIDUAL OR MULTI VITAMINS

While individual vitamins are a great way to restore any depletions of specific nutrients in the body, the average child needs a more balanced dose of vitamins than individual vitamins can provide. In order for a child to get the vitamins needed, they would need to be given a vast number of individual vitamins each day. A multivitamin can provide a balanced dose of everything needed in one dosage. Another benefit of multivitamins is that there are many brands that are developed specifically for children. Individual vitamins are generally not made in doses appropriate for children, and can increase the likelihood of an overdose of a specific type of vitamin.

WHAT BRANDS ARE BEST?

There are many companies that currently make children's vitamins. Some are better than others. However, many doctors disagree on what is truly the healthiest and best type for children. Always compare the ingredients on the back of the container with the recommended dosages for children before purchasing a vitamin. Feel free to ask your doctor what brand may be best for your child's specific needs.

Many children just will not take vitamins that do not taste good! With this in mind, most doctors agree that it is best to give a child whatever vitamin that they don't mind taking. Many vitamins come complete with a child friendly appearance in shapes of cartoon characters. Finding a children's vitamin that your child will take without a battle each morning is the key to picking a brand of children's vitamins.

ENCOURAGING CHILDREN TO TAKE VITAMINS

It is important to encourage children to take their vitamins on a daily basis. Making vitamins a part of the daily breakfast routine is one way to encourage the proper intake. For children who do not like to take vitamins, a chart with a reward system is a great way to motivate them. Create a chart for the wall and allow the child to add a sticker each day after they take their vitamin. At the end of a week where they have consistently taken their vitamins allow them a reward, such as skipping dish duty for a night, or some sort of a small trinket.

It is also important to instill in children a sense of how important vitamins are in their health so that they will continue to take their vitamins as they get older. School based health programs often do a wonderful job at educating children on the importance of a balanced diet. This doesn't let you off the hook at home, though! Further stress the importance of vitamins to your children, even before they are school age. Set a good example for your children by taking vitamins yourself. Remember, children are curious creatures and sometimes giving them a rational for doing something (in this case taking vitamins) is much more effective than "because we said so."

AT WHAT AGE SHOULD CHILDREN TAKE VITAMINS?

As infants, babies that are breast fed gain a lot of their necessary vitamins through their mother's breast milk. For this reason, in addition to maintaining their own health, breastfeeding mothers should be sure to keep an adequate amount of vitamins in their own systems. It is also important for breastfeeding mothers to remember that the daily vitamins needed for a baby is different than what an adult needs. In order to avoid giving infants a dose of vitamins that may be too large, ask your physician if there are any foods or vitamin supplements that you should not ingest while breastfeeding. Not all vitamins pass through a mother into her breast milk, so the remainder of vitamins you need should be gained through external sources.

Because most children's vitamins are chewable, vitamins should be started in toddler hood. Until this age, it is twice as important to make sure that the child's food sources have the necessary vitamin intake.

Ask a doctor for an idea of what children should be eating to ensure they receive all of their nutritional needs. Babies who are fed baby formula need the type of formula that is rich in vitamins. Doctors can recommend a good formula that is right for your baby's needs. This is somewhat different from child to child. Babies with milk allergies who are fed with soy formulas may require additional vitamins not available in their formulas.

WHAT VITAMINS SHOULD BE AVOIDED IN CHILDREN?

As long as the child does not have any specific health problems, there are really no single vitamins that should not be given to a child. Multivitamins that are formulated for children have been designed to incorporate exactly what a child needs to grow and develop in a healthy manner. For some children with particular ailments , it may be best to avoid some vitamins. If your child has any kind of health problems, it is important to ask a doctor for advice before giving your child any vitamin supplements. Vitamins can also interact with some medications, so if your child is being prescribed any type of medications due to illness, ask the prescribing physician if you should hold off on their multivitamin while the medication is being administered. Always make sure your child's doctor knows what vitamins your child is taking on a day to day basis.

Some parents who worry about finicky eaters worry that their child may not be getting adequate nutritional needs even through vitamins, and wonder if it is a good idea to give additional vitamins to their picky eaters, or double dosing on vitamins in weeks that a child has had a particularly poor diet. This is absolutely not the case, as children's multivitamins are formulated for exactly the amount a child needs. It is a bad idea to give a child additional vitamins unless directed to do so by a doctor, even if the child has not been eating well.

3

VITAMINS, MEDICATIONS,

AND HEALTH BENEFITS

VITAMINS AND MEDICATIONS

Vitamins are an important nutritional resource, and for this reason doctors may prescribe certain vitamins specific to one's own needs. One example of this would be the prescription of folic acid and other prenatal vitamins to pregnant and nursing mothers. In addition to this, there are some medications prescribed for certain ailments that actually deplete the levels of vitamins in the body. Doctors will prescribe vitamins in conjunction with some medications, but some vitamins actually counteract the affects of medications. That's why it is important to avoid some vitamins when taking certain medicines. Ask a doctor about your vitamin intake when being given a new prescription.

POSSIBLE INTERACTIONS WITH MEDICATIONS

When taking some medications, certain vitamins should be avoided. Some medications used for treatment of acne and skin problems can interact poorly with Vitamin A. These medications increase the risk of Vitamin A toxicity and for that reason, the vitamin should not be taken. Vitamin B-6 should be avoided when taking prescription Levodopa. However, when Levodopa is taken in conjunction with Carbidopa, the concern of vitamin B-6 interactions is eliminated. For this reason, most doctors now prescribe both medications together.

Warfarin is a medication that is known to have negative side effects when taken simultaneously with vitamin E. Some studies have shown that some people taking both Warfarin and vitamin E have an increased risk of internal bleeding which can lead to serious health complications. Warfarin should also not be taken with Vitamin K, as the vitamin K can decrease the effectiveness of the Warfarin.

Phenytoin is a medication known to interact with folic acid. This is not a common problem, because most over-the-counter folic acid pills are not given in high enough doses to interact with Phenytoin. It is still important, however to check with your doctor when being prescribed Phenytoin before you takefolic acid. Because senior citizens generally take multiple medications, it is always very important to consult a doctor about what medications are safe to take.

VITAMINS THAT BOOST THE EFFECTS OF MEDICATIONS

Some medications have been found to be more effective when given in conjunction with certain vitamins. One example of this is Vitamin D. Medications that are prescribed to help with bone health are actually given a boost in efficiency by Vitamin D. Vitamin D is also shown to help with medications that help fight osteoporosis. Some studies show that vitamin D along with magnesium helps with the development of bone in teenage girls.

The B complex vitamins have been shown to boost the affects of medications that help with brain development and muscle and body development. Vitamin E is used in conjunction with immune system boosting medications, especially in the elderly.

HEALTH BENEFITS TO SENIOR CITIZENS

Seniors have specific needs in order to stay healthy. As people get older, they generally develop greater health needs, have a less efficient immune system, and become more fragile in structure. Due to their specialized needs, it is especially important for senior citizens to maintain an adequate supply of vitamins in their diets.

CALCIUM AND BONE DENSITY

Calcium is a very important part of nutrition, especially in senior citizens. When a person reaches the age of seventy, their bones can become quite brittle. To help combat this, calcium supplements can be taken. Few people realize that an adequate amount of calcium is not in the diet of the average person. In the human body, two percent of the body's weight is actually made up of calcium, almost all of which is found in the teeth and bones.

A calcium supplement should be a part of the daily routine for the elderly, especially with women who are prone to osteoporosis, a word which literally translates to "porous bones". Each year, about twenty percent of the body's calcium is destroyed and replenished through food and supplements. A person stands to lose a good deal of their bone health pretty quickly if they are not sufficiently taking in the calcium they need regularly.

While calcium is necessary and should not be ignored, it is not a good idea to take more of it than recommended. Anything above the required amount of calcium has no additional benefits to the body. When the recommended amount has doubled it actually can have side effects and can cause sickness.

BENEFITS OF FIBER

Fiber is a form of carbohydrates that are not broken down and digested by the body. Instead, fiber is excreted from the body in the feces. There are two different types of fiber, called soluble and insoluble. When mixed with liquid, soluble fiber forms a gel like substance, and binds with fatty acids. Soluble fiber lowers cholesterol, reducing the risk of heart disease. It also helps to regulate blood sugar in individuals with diabetes. Insoluble fiber passes directly through the intestines and helps balance the pH levels of the intestines, which helps prevent colon cancer. Insoluble fiber promotes regular bowel movements and prevents constipation, and removes toxic waste from the colon in less time.

Fiber intake is usually broken down into seventy-five percent insoluble fiber and twenty-five percent soluble fiber. It is recommended that the average person gets twenty-five grams of fiber each day. Fiber can be acquired by eating oats, bran, nuts, seeds, barley, and some vegetables. It's important to make sure your diet contains enough fiber to keep your body working the way it should. Because the elderly often do not get enough fiber in their diet however, it is a good idea to take a fiber supplement. Fiber supplements come in both pill form and powder form, which is dissolved into a liquid.

SUPPLEMENTS TO BOOST MEMORY

Over time, pollutants can build up in the brain and impair memory function. These pollutants can come from habits such as smoking and drinking, or simply being exposed to such things as air and water pollution. The older people get, the more their memory can be impaired by this. There are many vitamins on the market that will help to prevent this problem, and when you are taking the proper amounts of them, your brain and memory function can be improved.

The B Vitamin groups, especially folic acid, and Vitamins B-6 and B-12 help with brain function. They are especially helpful with information processing, and verbal skills. This is an important group of vitamins for the elderly, whose brain function begins to slow down. Vitamin B-6 has been proven to help with memory retention, and the other B vitamins have been shown to promote mental clarity. Each different B vitamin helps in a slightly different way, but almost all of them are quite necessary with the development of the brain and brain function.

By taking their B vitamins, the elderly are helping to keep their minds and bodies strong for years to come.

Vitamin E has been shown to help improve memory function by neutralizing the chemicals that are collected in the brain over time by cigarette smoke, alcohol, and air pollution. Taking Vitamin E can be especially helpful in trying to help with the memories of those who have led particularly unhealthy lifestyles. Drugs, cigarettes, and alcohol consumption often times help contribute to memory loss down the line, because these pollutants deposit into the brain and cause problems with brain development and functioning, as well as memory functioning.

Vitamin C helps with brain function as well, and aids in the overall lifetime performance of memory and other brain functions. Some studies have even shown that those who receive an adequate supply of vitamin C even have a tendency to live longer lives. Vitamin C is especially important in the elderly who tend to have less adequate immune systems than those whom are younger. Vitamin C helps boost the immune system and keep the elderly healthy as they get older.

DOCTOR RECOMMENDED VITAMINS AND SUPPLEMENTS

Due to declining bone health in most elderly people, it is important to always take a calcium supplement and maintain an adequate supply of calcium in the body to help prevent brittle bone disease and broken bones due to falls. It is also quite important to take a daily fiber supplement because it is unusual for an elderly person to ingest all of the necessary fiber that is needed to keep one healthy simply from diet alone. Because the elderly are less likely to be exposed to prolonged sunshine, a Vitamin D supplement is also recommended, especially since it can also help with bone density and bone strength. In fact, the required amount of Vitamin D is greater in an elderly person than a person of a younger age.

Folate and Vitamin B-12 are vitamins that are also greatly recommended for seniors. These will aid in both digestion and proper skin health. Luckily, most multivitamins that are designed for seniors aim their content directly to what most seniors are said to need. Shopping for vitamins based upon who will be taking them is a fairly simple and fool proof method of deciding how much of each vitamin and mineral is needed for that individual person. Of course, consulting a doctor on which multivitamin or single vitamin is best for a particular person can give one a better insight on what is perfectly right for them.

4

VITAMINS AND MEN

VITAMINS MEN NEED

All people have different nutritional needs. These needs are based on physiology, and are therefore very different between men and women. In an attempt to design exactly what is needed for them, some males turn to men's multivitamins. Others try to take separate supplements of exactly what they feel they need. In either scenario, it is important to develop a healthy balance between supplemented vitamins and a healthy diet.

MEN'S MULTIVITAMINS

If one is not inclined to try to create their own cocktail of vitamins and supplements, there are a number of multivitamins out there on the market designed specifically for men. These vitamins range in both price and efficiency, however one does not necessarily correlate to the other. In other words, the most expensive products are not always the best.

The best way to determine a good vitamin is to read the ingredients on the back of the bottles while you are out shopping. Compare which packages contain more essential vitamins and nutrients. A word of caution is necessary here. While cost does not necessarily indicate a good vitamin, exceptionally cheap supplements are generally created from synthetic nutrients and are therefore not as healthy for you. Synthetic nutrients are not as easily processed by the body, and therefore are less effective.

The most effective way to choose a good multivitamin is to speak with your doctor and see what he or she recommends.

Some doctors will even direct you toward prescription vitamins that may be balanced better for you, and could even be covered by insurance.

VITAMINS AND SUPPLEMENTS TO INCREASE SEX DRIVE

There are many drugs on today's market to help increase a male's sex drive. However, there are even more products on the market that consist of natural vitamins and herbal supplements that can accomplish much the same thing. By taking natural supplements to accomplish an increase in libido instead of artificial products, one is able to achieve the same desired result without polluting the body with the unnatural substances found in other drugs.

Vitamin A is one vitamin that helps contribute to a man's sex drive. Because Vitamin A works with the synthesis of progesterone, it is directly linked to a man's sex drive. Vitamin A deficiency is actually a common cause of male impotence.

Vitamin B is as aforementioned not truly a vitamin, but a hormone. This hormone works with the nervous system, and when it is taken in the recommended dosages can actually increase the sensitivity males encounter.

Vitamin C is not only essential in helping the development of many hormones that affect the sex drive, but also essential in helping with fertility. Men who maintain an adequate intake of vitamin C are less likely to have fertility problems than those who do not.

Zinc is one of the key components in testosterone and sperm production. A man who is lacking in zinc may be experiencing a vast array of problems in the bedroom. Zinc helps to create sperm and maintain the volume of semen in the body.

MEN'S HERBAL SUPPLEMENTS

In addition to vitamins, herbal supplements such as ashwagandha, ginger, cloves, gingko, horny goat weed, maura puama, yohimbe, and zallouh root are a very well known to increase a man's sex drive and sperm production.

- **Ashwagandha** is an herb similar to ginseng. It is known for helping to cure impotence and infertility. This herbal supplement increases both sexual desire, and the production of sperm.

- **Ginger/Cloves/Gingko** all help fight against impotence. These herbs all act in similar ways. One way is by increasing the blood floor to the extremities of the body, and the other is by acting as a warming agent to the body as well.

- **Horny goat weed**, though interestingly named, has been a celebrated herb of Chinese herbalists since prior to the birth of Christ. This is used in men to treat impotence, increase sperm production, and increase sexual energy.

- **Maura Puama** is another herbal supplement known to help with impotence problems. In addition to this, Maura Puama is an aphrodisiac that works in both men and women alike.

- **Yohimbe** is exceptionally affective for increasing libido and for assisting with erectile problems. However, it does not come without a price. as Yohimbe is also known for causing headaches and dizziness. This is not the case for all men, however, and the positive effects of yohimbe are almost instant, so it may be worth a try.

- **Zallouh Root** is somewhat hard to find and can be moderately expensive because it only grows in very specific mountain regions. For those men that have access to it or don't mind paying the price, zallouh root has been used for years in treating erectile dysfunction and increasing sexual desire.

VITAMINS AND SUPPLEMENTS MEN SHOULD AVOID

While some vitamins are especially good for men, others are equally as bad. Doctors and experts will recommend certain vitamins and supplements and will also alternatively recommend avoiding others as well. Some of the vitamins and supplements that should be avoided include liquid creatine, chitosan, L-carnitine, pyruvate, and ribose. As for herbs, licorice (including the black licorice candy), dong quai, fennel, hops, peony, and white willow should all be avoided.

It is important to always properly research any herbal supplement or vitamin supplement you are thinking of taking before purchasing it. Herbal experts are great resources for developing your knowledge of herbal supplements. Doctors can also be consulted, though knowledge of herbs varies from doctor to doctor, as does their opinions on herbs vs. medications. When all else fails, books and the Internet are great ways to do your own research on the specific herb you are questioning. No herb should ever be taken without first doing the proper research, so do not ever jump right into an herb because you have "heard good things about it."

HERBAL SUPPLEMENTS TO AVOID

- **Licorice** is one herb that should be absolutely avoided by men who are trying to impregnate their partners. Licorice, though known to increase the sex drive, also causes a decrease in sperm count. This does include the candy black licorice!

- **Dong quai** is an herb common to women's treatments. For every ounce of effectiveness it has for women it has equal parts of problematic effects for men. This herb helps to increase estrogen and can upset the natural balance of a man's body.

- **Fennel** is another herb that is great for women by counteractive to men. While the herb will increase the sex drive of a woman it will actually decrease libido in a man and should therefore be avoided.

- **Hops** is another herbal supplement that men should avoid. Although helpful for the treatment of minor ailments hops has a nasty side effective of decreased libido and even impotence.

- **Peony** is taken usually in root form. It's one more herb that's greatly helpful for regulating women's menstrual symptoms but devastating to the male libido. In addition, peony can be quite toxic if not taken correctly and in proper dosages, so should always be avoided unless an herbal expert has been consulted.

- **White willow** is the natural basis for the synthetic base to aspirin. This gift from nature has wonderful aspirin like effects such as decreasing pain and reducing fever. It also raises estrogen levels and can cause sexual dysfunction in men.

OTHER SUBSTANCES TO AVOID

- Some doctors will advise that **creatine** is a great substance for assisting in muscle development, while other doctors disagree and state that it is unnatural and unhealthy for the body. For those that do desire to take this supplement, the liquid form is one that should be avoided. Liquid creatine in studies has shown that they have no greater affect than a placebo. Some claim that the liquid form is more readily accepted into the body, but there is nothing scientific to back up these claims.

- **Chitosan** is a supplement that claims to work as a fat blocker. There are no proven scientific studies that have shown this to be the case. What studies have shown, however is that chitosan can cause gastric disturbances and other unpleasant health problems. This supplement should just be generally avoided.

- **L-Carnitine** is claimed by some to give increased energy and foster weight loss. In regards to claims of increased energy, there is simply no scientific research to back up these claims. As far as the weight loss is concerned, some studies have shown L-Carnitine to promote weight loss; however there are significantly more studies that have shown that it does not.

- **Pyruvate** is supposed to cause weight loss by increasing ones metabolism. While this is the case, it is only true when you are taking a massive dose of pyruvate (approximately 350 pills a week). In order to have pyruvate stimulate weight loss, you would be required to take what is a potentially toxic dose of the substance.

- **Ribose** is sold with claims of increasing energy. No studies have ever been conducted to back this claim up. This is yet another supplemental product that probably has no positive effects in the area it claims to.

5

VITAMINS AND WOMEN

VITAMINS WOMEN NEED

Like children, senior citizens, and men, women have specialized needs in their vitamin intake. Vitamins should be taken that help them not only to stay healthy, but also to help balance out their natural menstrual cycles. Many people would be amazed to know how greatly vitamins and herbal supplements can help with the female reproductive system, from relieving pre-menstrual symptoms to increasing sex drives, right down to helping with conception.

EXTRA AMOUNTS WOMEN NEED

Women need a lot of the same daily vitamins as their male counterparts. There are four vitamins and two minerals that women need especially. Vitamin E, Vitamin K, and Magnesium are three of the vitamins that are especially needed in women. In addition to these three vitamins, it is important for breastfeeding women to also take zinc each day. Calcium and Iron are two very important minerals that women should remember to consume daily as well.

WOMEN'S MULTIVITAMINS

Some women try to take individual vitamins each day, while others prefer to get their daily requirements by taking one simple pill. For these women, specialized women's vitamins are the way to go. Women can also talk to their doctor to see if any prescription or over-the-counter vitamins are recommended.

For females who are trying to become pregnant, are pregnant, or are nursing, specialized prenatal vitamins are both recommended and encouraged. These are available both with a prescription and over-the-counter. Prescription vitamins often come with the added bonus of being covered by insurance. Prenatal vitamins are an important part of making sure your baby develops in a healthy way. Women carrying babies who are depleted of vitamins have a much higher risks of having babies born with health problems – for instance, Spina Bifida is a devastating life-long disability caused by pregnant mothers not getting enough folic acid.

Do not be fooled into thinking one brand of vitamin is better than another simply because it costs more money, as this is not always the case. Always remember to keep in mind what types of vitamins and minerals your multivitamin should have in it, and compare that to the ingredients listed on the bottle. Pay special attention to the amount of each vitamin and mineral listed on the bottle, and compare that to what is the recommended daily dose.

VITAMINS TO INCREASE THE SEX DRIVE

There are a number of vitamins and herbal supplements that women can take to increase their sex drive. Aphrodisiacs are found quite readily throughout nature, both in herbal, vitamin, and mineral form. The vast amounts of these supplements that are available should be able to cover most any problem a woman may have in the bedroom. While medications to deal with the female libido are around and available, they are not nearly as well researched as the male versions. In many ways, women are better off finding natural ways to deal with their desires, or lack thereof.

- **Vitamin A** is often used in conjunction with the female libido. The vitamin contributes to the production of estrogen, and therefore helps a woman feel a little more sexually driven. Daily doses of vitamin A are said to really increase a woman's sex drive.

- **Vitamin B**, a hormone and not truly a vitamin, works by increasing levels of arousal. This happens because Vitamin A makes the body more sensitive to touch and other sensations, due to its affecting the nervous system.

- Vitamin C is great for women who want to increase their sex drive and their fertility. Vitamin C also decreases the likelihood of women getting sick, and healthy women are much more likely to have a full sex drive.

- **L-Arginine** is an amino acid that has major affects to the libido of a woman, and her partner as well. An L-Arginine supplement can be as effective for women as prescription drugs and is widely encouraged throughout the globe.

WOMEN'S HERBAL SUPPLEMENTS

There are some herbs that are beneficial to both genders in terms of the health of their reproductive systems. Most are beneficial to both men and women. Herbal supplements that have positive effects on women include ginseng, fo-ti, Damiana, Tongkat Ali, and Maca.

- **Ginseng** serves as a natural aphrodisiac and in fact, is one of the best selling herbs on the market. This herb is also credited with giving increased brain function and concentration. Ginseng is quite safe and effective, but of course should only be taken within its recommended dosages.

- **Fo-ti** is a Chinese herb that has been used for centuries to increase a woman's libido. While this supplement is also used for men, it seems to have more profound effects on women than on their partners.

- **Damiana** is another herb that is known to be a wonderfully successful aphrodisiac. This plant has been used in Mexico for years for this very purpose, and in more recent years has made its way to other countries for the same reason.

- **Tongkat Ali** is an herb known for increasing libido in both men and women. This herb comes from Malaysian countries and in its own region is actually more popular than prescription medications!

- **Maca** dates back to ancient civilization. It is credited to increased physical strength as well as a heightened libido. Maca has been taken for many years as a way of naturally boosting an individual's sex drive.

VITAMINS AND SUPPLEMENTS WOMEN SHOULD AVOID

HERBS WOMEN SHOULD AVOID

Some herbs area not healthy for a woman to take, especially if she is nursing, pregnant, or thinks she may become pregnant soon. While herbs are all natural, they not all healthy, and some of them can be quite harmful. It's important to thoroughly research any herb or supplement before taking it to insure that it will have only the most positive effects on your health.

Herbs that should be avoided by women at all cost include Black cohosh, blue cohosh, pennyroyal, ginger, dong quai, licorice (yes ladies, this does include the candy!) and fenugreek. These herbal supplements have a variety of side effects that can be devastating to the woman's body, especially a pregnant woman.

• **Black cohosh** is occasionally used under the direction of an experienced herbalist, doctor, or midwife, in order to encourage contractions and labor toward the end of a pregnancy. If it is taken any earlier than this in any amount, can cause a miscarriage.

• **Blue cohosh**, like its brother herb, should also never be taken in an quantity during pregnancy, for fear of causing contractions which could lead to early labor and miscarriage.

• **Pennyroyal** is an herb that can cause hemorrhaging and death in a pregnant woman. Like Cohosh, it can also cause contractions and in fact, was even given throughout history in large doses to women in order to make them abort.

- **Ginger** is a great herb to alleviate nausea and flu like symptoms, however during pregnancy can actually case birth defects to the unborn child much like the use of drugs can. Ginger should be avoided both during pregnancy, and during conception.

- **Dong quai** is yet another herb that can cause premature uterine contractions along with birth defects, and therefore should be avoided prior to conception as well as throughout pregnancy.

- **Licorice** and its black candy (the red varieties do not contain actual licorice) can be very aggravating for those trying to conceive. Licorice decreases the likelihood of conception and also increases blood pressure.

- **Fenugreek** is in line with the above mentioned herbs. This herb also causes uterine contraction during pregnancy which can easily lead to miscarriages and should be strictly avoided in pregnant women.

OTHER SUPPLEMENTS WOMEN SHOULD AVOID

Herbs are not the only supplements that should at times be avoided by women. Some supplements should be avoided at all times by women while other supplements only need to be avoided before and during pregnancy and while breastfeeding. Some of the more common supplements that women should avoid include, but are not limited to, vitamin A, vitamin D, and alfalfa.

- **Vitamin A** is an important part of health, but when more than 10,000 IU of this nutrient is taken daily by a pregnant women, it can severely increase the rate and likelihood of birth defects. Please consult a doctor if you are pregnant or nursing and you think your daily intake of vitamin A is greater than 10,000 IU.

- For the same reason, **vitamin D** should not fall outside of the guidelines of 400-1,000 IU each day. Anything lower than 400 IU can cause the pregnant mother to be unhealthy, but anything over 1,000 IU a day creates a chance to cause birth defects.

- Women who are presently taking birth control pills, blood thinners, aspirin, Warfarin, Heparin, or potassium should not take **alfalfa supplements**. The risks and complications with alfalfa combined with any of the above mentioned substances can be quite severe including severe bleeding. Birth control is also much less affective when alfalfa is taken and there is an increased risk of pregnancy.

It is quite important for any woman who is thinking of taking any type of vitamin or other supplement to speak with their doctor before taking it, especially if they are breastfeeding, pregnant, or trying to become pregnant. Precaution certainly outweighs trying to correct whatever problems could be caused by taking the wrong thing.

6

SUPPLEMENTS VS. FOOD

GETTING VITAMINS THROUGH FOOD

There is plenty of debate among nutritional experts over whether or not vitamins should be primarily attained through food or through vitamin supplements. Those in favor of food feel that it is a more natural way to get their required daily vitamins. The experts who lean toward supplements feel that they are a more accurate way to ensure good health. In truth, the answer is probably somewhere in between these two extremes. It is important to eat a healthy and balanced diet, but because preparing a diet that is one hundred percent nutritionally balanced would take nearly as long as a full time job, supplementing through vitamins is great idea as well.

ADVANTAGES OF A BALANCED DIET

Eating a balanced diet is quite important, regardless of whether or not a person takes supplements. The body requires more than just vitamins to stay healthy, and the natural balance that fruits, vegetables, proteins, and carbohydrates provide to the body is essential to healthy living.

Those who eat a balanced diet are shown to be in better physical condition, have fewer health problems, feel more energized, have a stronger immune system, and live longer lives than those who are less cautious about what goes on their plates. It's important to balance ones diet so that the body is supplied with the correct amounts of vitamins, minerals, and proteins, and eating healthy is a great way to begin this process.

DISADVANTAGES OF VITAMINS THROUGH DIET

Getting your vitamins and nutrients from your diet is a wonderful way to help keep your body happy and healthy. However, it is nearly impossible to receive all of the necessary essentials simply from eating right. Almost no one eats right all of the time, even when they are making a conscious effort to do so. Even when meals are perfectly balanced, they do not always contain the vitamins and minerals that they are thought to have.

Most people do not realize that cooking foods vastly breaks down their vitamin content, significantly reducing their nutritional value. The process of heating the food breaks down the vitamins structure. When we eat cooked food, it ends up having not even half of the assumed nutritional intake as one would expect. It is for this reason that eating cooked food leaves one at a disadvantage if they are trying to pack all of their daily nutritional needs into their diet alone.

This is also important to keep in mind that when dealing with children. it's especially difficult to keep a child eating only the healthiest foods and able to receive proper nutrition from their diet alone.

ARE ALL VITAMINS AVAILABLE IN FOOD?

To put it simply; yes. All vitamins are available in food. However, it is often nearly impossible to get the required daily dose of them through food alone. The recommended doses of some vitamins would require vast amounts of foods in order to hit the minimum required amounts, and that is only taking into account one vitamin.

The human body requires many vitamins each day, all with a certain amounts that need to be met throughout the day. It is virtually impossible to develop eating habits that incorporate the entire required vitamin intake for each vitamin, so while yes, the vitamins are theoretically available in food, no, they are not always available in the correct amount.

HOW MUCH OF WHAT SHOULD I EAT?

This is the age old question of the food pyramid. It has been taught to children in school health classes for years now, and has become quite popular with the adults as well over more recent years. Though the food pyramid has made mild changes over the years with shifts in opinion of what exactly is needed, the prevailing model states the new recommendations.

The new model recommends that carbohydrates should be consumed in six to eleven servings each day. Fruits should include two to four servings, and vegetables should include three to five servings. Climbing higher up the pyramid, the dairy group as well as the protein group requires two to three servings each. At the top of the pyramid are fats, oils, and sweets, which are suggested to be used sparingly.

GETTING VITAMINS THROUGH SUPPLEMENTS

First and foremost, it is quite important to understand that taking daily supplements does not replace eating a healthy balanced meal. Just because one takes their vitamins does not mean that they can eat fast food and sweets as their primary food source. As with most things in life, it is important to attain a balance between the different dynamics.

Supplemented vitamins are not all the same across the board. They should be individually evaluated for both health benefits and efficiency. It's also a good idea to discuss with your doctor what is recommended for you specifically. Anyone who is taking any medications should also consult their doctor in case of rare but potentially harmful interactions.

WHAT IS THE ADVANTAGE?

The main advantage to getting your vitamins from a supplement is that your body is able to expect and predict what nutrition it will have every day. The food that people eat each day is varied from meal to meal and therefore provides different nutrients each day, leaving the body in limbo not knowing what to expect. By taking a daily supplement the body is more naturally balanced.

Another great advantage of taking daily vitamins is the knowledge that even if your nutrition slips a little bit one day your body is still nourished with its daily requirements of vitamins and minerals.

WHAT ARE THE DISADVANTAGES?

There are really no real disadvantages in taking multivitamins when you do so in a smart and sensible way. A possible disadvantage would be consuming and relying on multivitamins that are not nutritionally sound. Another disadvantage would be relying only on supplements without eating a proper diet. However, as discussed earlier, these are all things that need to be maintained in conjunction with vitamin intake.

ARE ALL REQUIRED VITAMINS AVAILABLE AS SUPPLEMENTS?

Yes! When perusing the shelves of a local nutritional and health store, you will see that there are many manufactured supplements for all of your vitamin, mineral, and herbal needs. These vitamins can be purchased separately to create a blend of exactly what vitamins you feel are necessary in your system, but there is really no need for this. You will find that most multivitamins are actually proven quite effective in developing a nutritionally balanced blend for you.

MULTIVITAMINS OR INDIVIDUAL PILLS?

It is not recommended to simply blindly pick individual supplements and combine them without the proper research and recommendations from doctors, herbalists, or health specialists. An incorrect blend of supplements can disrupt the natural balance of the body, so when choosing individual vitamins, chose carefully!

In most cases, herbalists and nutritional specialists can be found in your local yellow pages. They would be happy to set up a time with you to discuss your daily activities and nutrition, and then evaluate what supplements would be best for you. A doctor can always be consulted about vitamin needs as well, though it is important to check with your doctor regarding his knowledge of herbal supplements. Not all doctors feel that they know every little detail about modern medicine.

LIQUID OR PILL FORM?

Newer studies have recently shown that liquid forms of vitamins or gel caps are more effective and more easily digested than the pill form. Allegations have even been made that the pill forms of some vitamins don't dissolve and digest in the body. No scientific studies have proven this idea, and many supplements are not available in liquid form. At present time, the jury is out on this question. However, some suggest that a liquid or liquid gel form is preferable when available.

7

A COMPREHENSIVE BREAKDOWN OF VITAMINS AND SUPPLEMENTS

In an attempt to understand what each vitamin consists of and how it affects the body, this chapter will outline various vitamins and their benefits on the body.

VITAMIN A

Vitamin A is from the retinoid group that helps with many functions of the body. This is found in many forms. The retinoid is broken down into alcohols in the small intestine before it is digested by the body.

WHY IS VITAMIN A NEEDED?

Vitamin A is needed for healthy vision through retinal formation, healthy skin through retinoid formation, and gene transcription by retinoic acid. The recommended dose varies based on age ranging from six hundred ULs daily for infants to 3000 ULs in lactating women between nineteen and fifty.

WHERE IS IT NATURALLY ACQUIRED?

Vitamin A is acquired naturally through liver, carrots, broccoli leaves, pumpkin, collard greens, papaya, sweet potatoes, eggs, kale, and many other foods. These foods vary in their content of vitamin A and are sometimes depleted of this source through cooking.

POTENTIAL FOR TOXICITY

Vitamin A is very rarely toxic because it must be taken in exceptionally high doses to become toxic. In a case of an overdose, vitamin A can cause vomiting, blurred vision, headaches, muscles and abdominal pain, weakness, drowsiness, and even an altered mental status.

Prolonged exposure to high doses of vitamin A can cause hair loss, fever, insomnia, weight change, brittle fractured bones, diarrhea, and the death of mucus membranes.

VITAMIN B

The B complex vitamins are actually eight vitamins that often coexist. They are all involved in cell metabolism. This group of vitamins includes thiamine, riboflavin, niacin, pantothentic acid, pyridoxine, biotin, folic acid, and cyanocobalamin.

WHY IS VITAMIN B NEEDED?

Vitamin B plays a vital role in controlling metabolism and increasing and supporting its rate It also helps in keeping the skin healthy, creating healthy muscle tone, encouraging cell division and cell growth, reducing the risk of some cancers, and enhancing the immune system as well as the nervous system.

WHERE IS IT NATURALLY ACQUIRED?

Vitamin B can be found in a variety of food sources, such as potatoes, chile peppers, liver oil, tuna, yeast, vegemite, and bananas. Each food contains a different level of vitamin B, and therefore does not contain equal content of B complex vitamins.

POTENTIAL FOR TOXICITY

In the rare case that Vitamin B is overdosed and toxicity occurs, some symptoms include numbness in the extremities, depression, low blood pressure, fatigue, hyperthyroid, migraines, heart palpitations, cramps, and much more.

With prolonged exposure, these symptoms significantly increase and can become detrimental to health and well being. Vitamin B only becomes toxic when it is taken many times above the recommended level, so illness can be avoided simply by following the recommended dosages.

VITAMIN C

Vitamin C is an essential nutrient that is found in most mammals. It is also known as L-ascorbate. It is still unclear how much Vitamin C is needed in the body to keep a person at optimal health. This number is being debated between specialists, some of whom believe adding extra Vitamin C to the body is quite helpful. Others feel that it has no affect.

WHY IS VITAMIN C NEEDED?

Vitamin C is a vital part of immune functioning. It is also essential in the healing of wounds and the strengthening of teeth. It's important to receive the recommended daily dose of Vitamin C in an attempt to fight off germs and viruses. Vitamin C helps to protect the body from many intruders by building the white blood cells in the immune system and readying them to fight off bacteria.

WHERE IS IT NATURALLY ACQUIRED?

Vitamin C perhaps the worst vitamin to try to ingest naturally through cooked foods. Most processes of food preparation destroy the natural vitamin C that foods have naturally within them. When food is prepared in a vitamin C conscious way however, it can be found in milk, liver, oysters, lamb, pork, and cod. Vitamin C can also be found naturally in fruits and vegetables such as grapefruit, raspberry, oranges, plums, pear, lettuce, eggplant, broccoli, parsley, and red pepper.

POTENTIAL FOR TOXICITY

Vitamin C is very difficult to overdose on because the amount of Vitamin C needed to consume to overdose is so high that most individuals would find it quite hard to consume. Signs of an overdose would be iron poisoning, kidney stones, diarrhea, and other flu-like symptoms.

As is the case with all vitamins, Vitamin C should only be taken as directed and within the recommended daily dose. While some believe that taking a mega dose of vitamin C to eliminate a cold is a great cure, scientifically, it has been proven that this does not work, and is even likely to cause illness.

VITAMIN D

Vitamin D is a prohormone that is used to maintain the organ system. There are two types of vitamin D, ergocalciferol and cholecalciferol, which is produced in the skin when exposed to sunshine.

WHY IS VITAMIN D NEEDED?

Vitamin D helps in a number of ways. It affects the immune system by acting as an anti-tumor agent. It inhibits the parathyroid hormone, and regulates the amount of calcium and phosphorus levels in the blood stream. Without the adequate amount of Vitamin D in the body, a person can develop a number of problems, such as rickets or osteomalacia.

WHERE IS IT NATURALLY ACQUIRED?

Sunlight is a great source of creating Vitamin D, however it is also found in milk, bread, margarine, butter, oil, yogurt, herring, catfish, salmon, eel, tuna, and sardines. The most important aspect of acquiring Vitamin D naturally is by making sure you get enough sunshine, because unless you spend a lot of time outdoors, normal day to day exposure to the sun is not sufficient for healthy Vitamin D creation.

POTENTIAL FOR TOXICITY

One is not at risk for Vitamin D overdose by prolonged sun exposure, only by consuming it naturally through foods, or in supplement form. Signs of Vitamin D toxicity include itchiness, increased urine production, renal failure, weakness, nervousness, nausea, and vomiting. If a Vitamin D toxicity is suspected, it is quite important to seek medical attention and discuss this concern with a doctor.

VITAMIN E

Vitamin E is a fat-soluble vitamin with properties of antioxidants. It is broken down into eight groups of tocopherals and tocotrienols. Vitamin E is essential to the body, and research is currently being conducted that seems to show it is beneficial in both preventing coronary heart disease and treating cancer. Vitamin E can be found naturally in the environment or taken in supplement form, where gel caps are readily available.

WHY IS VITAMIN E NEEDED?

Vitamin E is needed to regulate a lot of the body's natural symptoms. Some people are more prone to needing extra vitamin E, such as infants with low birth weights. There are even some genetic conditions that cause a depletion of vitamin E, requiring increased vitamin E consumption.

WHERE IS IT NATURALLY ACQUIRED?

Vitamin E can be acquired naturally from a variety of good sources. Wheat germ, almonds, asparagus, avocado, seeds, olives, and nuts are only a few of the many sources of Vitamin E.

POTENTIAL FOR TOXICITY

Though a vitamin E overdose is almost unheard of, it is thought by some experts that an exceptionally high dose of Vitamin E could cause bleeding. The FDA has not set a limit to the recommended dose of vitamin E because no side effects have been proven.

Printed by Libri Plureos GmbH in Hamburg,
Germany